The Sun Never Sets

Nathan Bowker

Introduction

I wrote a life story called Tomorrow and from it I took ideas and expanded them into personal essays. This is my first book of essays and I'm working on many more. My next one is titled Darkness. These two don't really reflect subject matter. The life story is more about 'this is what I've been through' and tomorrow is the future. Darkness and The Sun Never Sets play off the idea of Tomorrow - the duration of time, but the subject matter in Darkness isn't anything darker than this. I write a lot about medical topics because I've spent the majority of my life searching for answers. I got to a point where I could string together both my understanding and new theories. It was time I wrote it all down to share my journey. I don't have a degree in anything medically related, so I could be wrong on some things. I write about things as I understand them. I often find myself in a loop of research where even the answers don't quench my curiosity.

Uninterrupted

I'm imagining a life that is fluid. All of my schooling and behaviors melding into older versions of myself. I could admire the maturity and lessons learned, always developing into a more advanced person. It's only a fantasy.

What happened with me was a lifetime of immaturity with many stops and restarts. I've never felt like I belonged to any part of it, but one of those stops stands out to me the most. I had adapted into an arrogant, entitled person during my high school years. I did whatever I wanted: I made jokes at the expense of others, I disrupted class, the world revolved around me. I didn't really mature the way an adult typically does and I continued living childishly into adulthood.

A doctor took me from that path shortly after high school. Had my life continued unchecked, I might not have ever gained enough insight to change. To me nothing was broken, therefore there was nothing to fix. I envy how seemingly little thought goes into an ordinary man's life. Whatever it is I'm living is filled with worry and self-doubt. That doctor probably didn't set out to crush my ego that day. He was only doing the job he was trained to do. During a routine physical he noted my testicles were about 1/8 the size of normal.

I'm sure every person I had ever laughed at, hurt or did wrong had wished for something terrible to happen to me. I was just sailing through life collecting what I felt the world owed me. I finished high school and thought making it that far without any health issues meant I'd escaped any possibility until end of life complications appeared.

Karma had other ideas though and showed up at a time when I was limping through life without the crutch I relied on for so many years. My former crutch was sitting in a classroom and making jokes to receive laughter, which inevitably was my medicine. I used crutches to medicate - none of us wanted to be in a classroom and I passed the time while having fun. Karma appeared and shot a rope through time, affecting me retroactively. It hit me in the moment and it guided my passage backwards to delve into my past. I was able to tether myself to it and explore the person I once was and look for reasons why. I processed the information of not being a man through the stages of grief. I wondered if maybe I did something to cause it. Once in grade school I bit into the end of a thermometer and the mercury spilled into my mouth. The school nurse and everyone made a big deal about it and had me wash my mouth out numerous times. Had I inadvertently caused a defect in my future development? I also got kicked in the groin once in the 6th grade. It was so hard my vision went black and I've wondered if that caused it.

At age 19 that doctor pointed out an anomaly and I sunk to a low point afterward. I was embarrassed and ashamed of his notes. I didn't want anyone to ever see them and I refused to sign waivers for future medical staff. Imagine how embarrassed you'd be to be seen naked by strangers, perhaps with a scar across your chest. You may try to shield it with your arm whenever possible. Most people have some amount of shame about their naked bodies. But imagine that fear multiplied because of a verified report of a disorder. Let's compound that fear because it concerns the genitals. Now, add to it a society that emphasizes balls to mean courage, strength, virility, manliness. My ego was disfigured that day. My newfound diagnosis interrupted life and forced me into hiding.

For 8 years I dealt with it by only having drunken sex. I had to be drunk and I preferred my partner to be as well. I felt either they wouldn't notice or remember and that alcohol was the only thing that allowed me to have a sex life. My naked body disgusted me.

A word I would become familiar with was dysgenesis. The *dys* means: word-forming element meaning "bad, ill; hard, difficult; abnormal, imperfect," from Greek dys-, inseparable prefix "destroying the good sense of a word or increasing its bad sense" [Liddell & Scott], hence "bad, hard, unlucky," from PIE root (and prefix) *dus- "bad, ill, evil" (source also of Sanskrit dus-, Old Persian duÅ¡- "ill," Old English to-, Old High German zur-, Gothic tuz- "un-"), a derivative of the root *deu- (1) "to lack, be wanting" (source of Greek dein "to lack, want").

Genesis means: Old English Genesis, first book of the Pentateuch, which tells among other things of the creation of the world, from Latin genesis "generation, nativity," in Late Latin taken as the title of first book of the Old Testament, from Greek genesis "origin, creation, generation," from gignesthai "to be born," related to genos "race, birth, descent" (from PIE root *gene- "give birth, beget," with derivatives referring to procreation and familial and tribal groups).

In my case, the phrase I would learn to read about my condition described me as having *testicular dysgenesis.* No matter how you look at it, it means bad creation. Try adding those feelings to your naked self. It wasn't an irrational fear or an idea I had conjured in my head and chose to believe. It is in the medical terminology. To not believe it would be irrational.

My official diagnosis came many years later because I had found a doctor willing to take my blood to analyze. A simple blood draw was all it took to yield results. I was told I had Klinefelter's Syndrome, which allowed me to further investigate myself and every word used to describe me. *Dysgenesis* is far from the only word whose roots are negative in their native language concerning my description. I might be welcomed and cared for by doctors who've taken a Hippocratic oath, but I am described among them in an uncaring way.

I use etymology to help me understand language. People with Klinefelter's Syndrome suffer from learning disabilities with a heavy emphasis on language. It must just be something to do with that part of the brain failing to mature is my guess. Learning about root words in their native languages has served as a sort of a secret decoder that has unmasked everything. I have resentments as if looking into the Matrix at all these familiar words with hidden meanings. All around nothing is what it seems. Words are chosen to describe without considering their impact on those affected. A man goes through normal development, while I have suffered abnormal development. Coming from Latin is *abnormis* meaning monstrous combined with Greek *anomalos* meaning "not even." Anomalous in English means deviating from normal. Together they form abnormal. My development is monstrously uneven and a deviation. I gave no consent to be described as such a monster.

I feel like the person dubbed the Elephant Man yet not quite a man because of the dysgenesis in the anatomy doctors use to declare a male from a female. What am I? I had impulse control issues that altered proper psychosocial development. I didn't make friends or assimilate smoothly. I self-medicated with humor and later drugs. I spent my school years in detention and more years in prison. Society separates the monsters like myself with punitive isolation where any aberration is sure to prosper. I've dealt with being broken among others who were also defective, so the rest of you could enjoy being normal, away from monsters. I can only imagine in the place you were how the definition of normal was constantly being refined. I bet even among the normal, someone was a deviation. You would always need a scapegoat in order to feel normal.

I'm still tethered to my diagnosis in the present and moving forward. I've reached acceptance to my condition, but not toward my body. I'm still in the grieving process. I'm not okay being naked. It's a humiliation for me and I have a constant sense of being inferior. In my younger years I had no problem being horny. My problem was in having sex. Now that I'm older, I don't use drugs anymore and I'm married, but the shame is still there. I'm often not horny for sex and instead prefer masturbation when it does appear. I can feel the dysgenesis as if my testicles are dead and I prefer that term over broken to describe the dysfunction. Broken, to me, implies pain that brought it to its state. I have no pain, but a feeling of emptiness. I cannot reproduce. I carry a void between my legs. I use testosterone, which is about the only thing that makes me horny and I sometimes resist it because I don't like who it makes me. I feel as a foreign host to this body. I'm more or less castrated without it. The dysgenesis bleeds inward making me broken-hearted over who I'm not.

In social settings I simultaneously pretend to be a man while trying to add to the conversation and keep an even flow. I struggle with what to say, being focused, showing proper facial expressions and interest. I often fail. Put that in the box of shame you carry around. Try meeting new people and carrying on mundane conversations while holding back all these burdens.

I wonder what it would be like to have a life where each moment went into creating something better, where happiness and self-esteem both existed. If I were normal the entire time from the womb onward, if all the right chemicals appeared at all the right times and were invested into producing an asset for the planet, I wonder who that person would be had he lived uninterrupted.

Introspection 1
*This is a series that spans the course of the book
offering reflections, theories, my inner voice.*

Maybe those of us with XX chromosomes are babied by nature, which causes us to be more caring and nurturing caregivers; perhaps we are predisposed. The easiness by nature that I'm referring to is during development. XX women start and finish as the same embryo, whereas those of us with a Y undergo a chemical transition. Women who carry an XY child during pregnancy often report sickness more so than when they carry females; his androgens are as high as they would be during puberty and it causes the women carrying them to get sick[1]. I would imagine that it affects the baby with a similar kind of sickness. For 6-8 weeks the development went a certain way then a change occurred that was so severe it caused illness in the host body. Trauma can and does happen when children are too young to remember and it affects them for a lifetime. Maybe that's why males seem so cold and callous at times. XX women don't go through that trauma in early development. It's only during puberty the XX person gets a monthly chemical dose, but they are more equipped to process pain and the ill effects by that age. XXY individuals, such as myself, experience effects of androgens neonatally, but possibly not as severe as the XY and the evidence is in the feminization in certain parts of the body. (Look up Klinefelter's Syndrome on an image search.)

---

[1] A unique way of looking at this is that he's priming her for what will happen to him, in the household, in about 13 years.

Walls and Closets

I've spent the better part of my life in the closet. My sexual urges and fantasies were hidden in shame. As far back as I can remember I've been fascinated by the idea of humiliation and being subservient to domineering women. I've had those fantasies throughout my life, even while I created and achieved other fantasies. I didn't try acting on them soberly until I was in my 30s.

I began having sex with men when I was 18. This led to a lot of shame and denial also. I wanted to be straight, but the fantasy and anticipation boiled over until I needed to quench my appetite. I thought I could just do it once and get it out of my system. Like seeing the Grand Canyon, I could make my pilgrimage and never really need to visit it again.

I thad intense thoughts doing it for probably a year and a half. After I did, I swore to never do it again. But I was getting another fix a few months later. It fixed me in a sense so that I could focus on being straight with a new fervor. My fantasies and acting on them became shorter in duration. I tried to manage the urges in order to not be gay. *I wasn't a fag!* There was so much negative connotation with that word while growing up. I wasn't as scared to suck a dick as I was being called a fag. Being that word was a lifestyle of disrespect, whispers, judgement. I knew all about it because I lived a privilege. I was privileged in that I was present while straight people discussed this or that guy being a fag. They would make jokes as if how one preferred to achieve orgasm defined him as a human. I've heard them tell me someone was gay as a precursor to me meeting them. They'd whisper it before the person showed up, *My friend Johnathan is gay.*

What if one day the cool people hated on anyone who didn't do it doggystyle? If you had sex another way, you wouldn't want to talk about it even if you enjoyed it more than doggystyle. You'd be on the receiving end of shame and judgment. What consenting adults prefer in the bedroom shouldn't open them up for abuse in any area of their life. Could you imagine if the people at work or your siblings found out you like doing it missionary and being discriminated against, laughed at, or refused invitations? You might even lie to stay in good graces because no one outside of your bedroom really knows and a little lie doesn't change the person you are.

I've been in many relationships with women where I've had to play defense about my past. I never felt at ease enough to admit what I like and try to build a relationship of exploration with my partner. I might have found many things I enjoyed if I had ever found a place to feel welcomed and accepted. I'd probably have a higher self-esteem as well. But no, my sexual interests were guarded and even my vanilla straight sexual life was closeted in the sense of body dysmorphia. I built walls and through my presentation as a straight man, I attracted others who came with walls built in: *walls beget walls*. I relied on alcohol to allow me to feel comfortable in order to have sex. I also needed alcohol to express my kinky desires and more alcohol to foster my sexual needs with men.

I wore the mask of toxic masculinity: if I talked negatively about fags then the logic was that I couldn't be one. So I spent several years as a troll and never found out who I was. I was a dichotomy between who I was socially vs sexually. By living two separate lives there was an identity that failed to mature in a healthy and positive way. It was who I could have been had I felt safe to nourish my soul and reach my full potential.

Instead, I've had to deny and sneak around to meet my needs. I started living soberly around age 30 and started exploring my kinkier, straight desires a few years after that. When I've met someone who is accepting of my desires, it's only for a few hours while I'm in their company. I wear my mask on my way to and from meeting up. I've gotten so used to my outwardly persona and the way I'm treated that I don't want to risk changing it. I'm not sure the benefit outweighs the risk.

It took me quite a few years to develop this appearance I present to the world. From first glance to first conversation, my sometimes stoic charm leaves a lasting impression. I stand 6'6" tall and almost 300 lbs. I have literally spent years sculpting my body into a muscular powerhouse and have been practicing longer than that in acting straight. It's quite a juxtaposition as I've rejected masculinity on so many other levels. I don't give a shit about sports or 4wd trucks, camping, hunting, etc. My body naturally rejects masculinity and it is only with the help of synthetic testosterone am I able to showcase my impressive physique. The biggest mirage is to the eyes of judgement: I probably bestow strength and virility. I was destined to spoil the dreams of whatever woman tried to get close enough for me to let down my walls and confide my true nature.

I'm submissive in my heart. I'm also into wearing clothes made for women. I desire playing the part of a woman either sexually or as a private lifestyle. Service oriented submission, that is, performing services such as cooking and cleaning turn me on in a sense. I seek to challenge the traditional gender binary and toy with role reversal. In addition I like deep, psychological games that taunt my arousal. I don't always need sex or to otherwise achieve an orgasm. I like being used and getting nothing in return. I crave certain types of pain and punishment that is meted out in ever crafty ways. All my potential to live a healthy life was stuffed into a box where my natural expressions felt sick and unhealthy. Still, I struggled to find ways to come out in the dark corners to express a sliver of myself before withdrawing again. Having parts of me that lived an inhibited self led to more creative ways to seek excitement. All the shame I buried myself in became the very thing I eroticized in safety.

I've lived a contradictory life and so I crave mind fuckery. I believe those two are related. I need role-play scenarios that exploit my vulnerabilities. I've feared not being masculine the most and through a kink lifestyle I'm able to face those fears. I endorse people telling me the most fucked up things possible that attack my "manhood." But the more I do it, the more relaxed I become and the more I need it. When no one is home, I prefer to wear a dress just to watch TV.

It's easy to read history and see how different societies discriminated against others. It's easy for most people to see how seemingly primitive past peoples behaved. We pass judgement on the times and appreciate the progress we've made. It's more difficult for people to apply those same lessons to current times and realize we are just as primitive as people have always been. People might swear to never do a disagreeable activity and label it *gay*. Each time the word gay is used negatively, it adds another barb to the wire - the word becomes a prison to those who try but can't change their sexuality. Bullies, friends and parents throw around the word fag so much that it is ingrained in us not be one. Even with religion in modern times, people who are empathetic to mankind often find ways to dehumanize gay men like they did in primitive times. The old adage: *Sticks and stones may break my bones, but words will never hurt me* is a lie. Words can become labels and your label becomes your brand and you have no choice what others think of the product you are. That brand becomes a branding which leaves its scar on your soul. I had become a fag and even while pretending throughout my life to be otherwise, I always knew deep down and I've wondered that maybe I don't deserve love because everything I've ever done is fake. The only time I've been real is when I sought out sex from men. I had nothing to hide from them. I feel at ease in their company. I don't have to hide that I like women when I'm with a man. Any man would take it as a compliment that I chose to be there with him despite my preference for women. If a woman had what I needed, why aren't I with her instead of there with him? Shame without acceptance is humiliation. With it, is humility.

When I was growing up, the only gay men I knew about were effeminate. I had a guy in high school and later met an older guy who was as well. I would have been more frightened to be like that because there would be no denying who I was. I wouldn't want that scar or try to represent that brand. I liked being me to the extent that I could secretly get my needs fulfilled while still performing for all eyes as a straight man. But then again, those effeminate men had more truthfulness and sincerity than I ever will. They were honest with themselves and didn't have to live the coward's life I chose.

My life has been a performance for the sake of others. I've lived a privilege based on deceit. As a result I've endured people's comments on gays when they thought no one was looking. I've unwillingly spied on the integrity of others and it has left a scar so deep that I cannot reconcile the damage. I am broken.

---

*I realize using the word *fag* is inflammatory. But I'm claiming/reclaiming it to take it out of the hands of inflammatory people.

We Are Not Pretty

I realize how inflammatory the title is, but I would like a moment to explain. I prefer women in my life over men. I like them as friends and lovers. I love the female form: the curves, eyebrows, long hair, eyelashes, makeup and nails. I love all shapes and body types. I also love being able to relate. I like their sensitivities and empathy, their compassion, the way they love.

I've spent most of my life chasing the attention and acceptance of women. I've spent several years proving I'm not a threat who was only trying to sleep with them. I genuinely sought to become friends. I wanted to be so close and not like other men, real men. *I'm not that kind of guy.* In the past women have said that very line about themselves: *I'm not that kind of girl.* Usually it was said to avoid some extreme sexual act that she was turned off by or as a means of playing coy.

For me, I use it to mean all sexual activity. I have body dysmorphia in a few areas including my genitals. My ego is shaped by the perception of others - I'm deeply afraid of their judgment. The world functions on: genitals = gender, and my genitals are ill formed, so what's that make me? Specifically, my testicles are lacking in size and performance. Our society equates balls as anything that is manly, courageous, virile, masculine. I'm not those things. I'm humble, docile, sensitive, scared.

For me to think, *I'm not that kind of guy,* it serves a few purposes. First it reinforces how I already feel. I don't want to fuck because I'm not a man. I don't want to lay on top of someone and thrust my pudet* until orgasm. It's not something I deserve to do. If that's all men want, then we *should* be friends. I have something she can't get from another male - that is a lack of wanting sex coupled with a sincere friendship. I'm just another female she can be friends with. I don't want sex because then she'd know what I have down there and that idea scares the daylights out of me. I'd rather she think of me as a girl, emasculating as that sounds, because I don't want her knowing what my genitals look like. Her psychological assumption would be easier for me to live with because there's always a shadow of a doubt: *maybe I am just a good friend.* If she knew definitively what I have down there I would feel more emasculated because there is no doubt of my physical deformity. If sex were involved, it would ruin our friendship and I'd have to try and be a man only to fail by appearance and perhaps, by performance. So it's much less emasculating to be treated as a girl than any of the alternatives. As a girlfriend I can just be me and succeed. Don't force me to be a man because: *I'm not that kind of guy.*

I've suffered with masculinity issues throughout most of my life. What does it really mean to be a man? I've tried using Google to come up with ideas. One thing I've never read on any list is a desire to wear dresses. Mmm, I love to wear a dress in the morning while drinking my coffee. I feel at peace to be a woman. All my conflict and failure dissipates. I'm not pretty in the sense of looking like the kinds of women I'm attracted to. I've spent a lifetime admiring women, either for sexual conquest in my younger years or the acceptance I now seek. I'm attracted by both beauty and intelligence. I'm a connoisseur of feminine radiance.

I went to an event where there were others like me, but who were openly expressing themselves. I was closeted, in my man clothes and looking through the crowd. It seems so ironic to be closeted at a kink event, dressed as the straight male I purport to be day in and day out. It's comparable to the idea that an undercover stripper has clothes on. How would you know they're a stripper while at a store? Equally, no one at the event knew any different than the costume I had on. I was a male to all eyes. I sat behind my mask and judged how unfeminine some of the trans women appeared. I scolded myself internally and decided I shouldn't continue my dressing because *we are not pretty.*

When I went home, I had confidence to explore the inner workings of my mind. The night had emboldened me. Just going and pretending to be the part of me who's unhappiest still put me there with the crowd. As soon as I got home I took some LSD I had been keeping in my refrigerator. I had been reluctant to take the plunge, mostly out of fear. I hadn't done LSD in over 20 years and I had had a few hits stashed in the refrigerator for a couple months trying to summon the courage. It wasn't even 30 minutes until I put a dress on. It didn't matter how I looked or how the women at the event looked. For me, it was about feeling. I felt like a woman and I felt at peace and that's all that mattered.

I think the success in appearance is better the earlier a person transitions from male to female. Ideally, they'd want to do it as early as possible in order to avoid the ill effects of testosterone. As an embryo, we all develop in the same way until about 6 weeks. At that point, those whose chromosomes are XY typically change course and become boys. If that process were delayed, a body could always masculinize later. I've seen pictures of adult women who used steroids for bodybuilding and they take on masculine features. Testosterone doesn't just target muscle tissue. It squares the jaw, creates facial hair, a deepening of the voice and their clitoris usually grows as if it were taking directions to become a penis. A woman transitioning to a male can basically do it at any time and see good results; it doesn't matter if it happens at 6 weeks or 36 years. They will become manly, but a man transitioning to a female has a tougher road to climb. All the masculinized effects he has undergone cannot be undone easily. You could always turn the Mona Lisa into one of Picasso's cubist renditions, but you cannot easily do the reverse. Round angles are easier to square than squares are to make round.

When I see a young transwoman who is as much feminine as the types of women I've fancied, I see a lot of strength. Her bravery is pretty. It's a difficult decision at any age, but it is exceptionally powerful to see her breaking from her prison early. The longer we stay, the more the well is poisoned by androgens. We may resist all through a grueling career, family life, perhaps waiting to outlive our parents in order to alter our canvas. Each year we postpone, we take on darker brush strokes, heavier masculine features and bone growth. We are imprisoned by what others may think, fear of our lack of beauty, being alone or unloved. We fear the unknown.

It's a race against nature to make such a decision. A developing teenager tends to make decisions based on emotion. They process information in their amygdala. Adults, on the other hand, make decisions using their prefrontal cortex. It's considered the rational part of the brain in that it takes into account past experiences, long-term consequences and overall good judgment. A person's brain isn't done connecting those two worlds until around age 25. So a male has been churning out testosterone for a solid 10+ years by that point. The race is to make such a decision both before the brain is fully developed and before testosterone causes unwanted effects. But, would a fully developed brain regret it later on? Is it a good decision if it's made in the amygdala? People who do it earlier are pretty in the sense of bravery and, by default, they enjoy a more of a feminine appearance, creating beauty physically, while those who do it later tend to be making a rational decision despite more pronounced masculine features.

I feel my story is different. I'm not sure changing my sex or gender expression publicly would help. I fear I'd still have a tough time fitting in regardless. I think my brain isn't right. I read body language and let the smallest things bother me. I can be as equally offended by what's not said as I would hearing an insult. If a coworker says goodnight to the guy next to me, but not me, then clearly he must not like me. Each day I go into situations where I worry there's negative judgment about me, and that's while living as a male. I wouldn't be able to cope as a female. It would be obvious that I used to be something I wasn't and am trying to be something I'm not.

The woman who's considered passable is an inspiration. Everyone wants to be attractive like her, but more than that, we seek to be free, *to be pretty*. No more pretending, trying to fill a role and failing.

*Pudet comes from Latin meaning causes shame

Introspection 2

What comes first: being M or being broken? If you're hypogonadic with a Y chromosome your body doesn't produce testosterone adequately, the organization in your brain isn't there. Your receptors haven't been primed and your genitals may not form properly. They might be present upon birth, so you can receive that M on your birth papers and you can grow up to be treated as M, using the M bathroom, and responses from others hold you to the idea of M. You're either encouraged or bullied into fulfilling your M statute. ...but you don't feel M underneath it all. All the evidence you gather on your own says it's not true, but now you have a lifetime built on lies. It's like you have to continue telling lies in order to keep the original lie. Who does that make you? The lie becomes a privilege to continue being treated as a normal M. It's like a hunter who doesn't understand what it's like not to be a hunter. They typically acquire the tradition from their fathers and pass it on to their sons. All around us people inherit customs and traditions ...it's only when you lose one do you realize the box you were once in.

I look at and study M behavior from the outside looking in. There are certain attributes in a person's life that scare me. If I deem them super masculine, I don't want anything to do with them. The other day in the store two guys wearing Carhartt gear asked me if I could give them a jumpstart. I was in my own Carhartt gear on my way to work. I must have appeared to them as a fellow brother; I appeared as a man they could relate to and they sought me out. I told him no and I left. I don't even know how to open my hood. I didn't want to have to fumble around with it in front of them. I wear Carhartt because people at work wear it. I had never even heard of the brand until I started working there. I wear it to blend in with men so no one doubts my lies.

Haunted Soul
This was written before *Tides*

I'm using this body as a shell so that my conscious being can exist and express itself while learning what this life offers. I didn't choose this vehicle or the time in history that I arrived and I'm not sure my journey would have been any easier had I arrived sooner. I suffer from hypogonadism. As a result of meager testosterone production I'm at great risk for a variety of health conditions. I don't know if it's by cause or effect, but I get respiratory illnesses quite often. It usually starts with nasal congestion and within a day or two it goes into my lungs. I've had bronchitis more times than I can count.

If I had shown up prior to the 20th century I wouldn't have access to a rescue inhaler. I typically need albuterol to keep my breathing issues in check once I start noticing difficulties. The aerosol inhaler wasn't patented for use until the mid 1950s. Sometimes I need a steroid inhaler in addition to help stabilize my breathing. Still, other times I go on to develop bronchitis. I've developed my own model for the stages of illness. 1. Denial: It might come on disguised as allergies; sinus congestion that moves into my lungs. 2. Bargain: I will bargain via my denial by using inhalers, allergy meds, honey, garlic whatever I can to remedy the situation quickly. 3. Irrationality: Once I realize that my bargaining is to no avail, I start looking at everything in my life with suspicion. Maybe I'm not drinking enough water, I need to change my sheets more, not play with the cats as much, stop drinking from BPA containers, take two showers a day to wash off pollen. I've even gotten to the point when I questioned whether the medicine I was taking was making me sick - the inhalers or Mucinex, etc. Finally I move toward acceptance and go see a doctor. The average time it takes me to get better from start to finish is 7 weeks. In 2019 I spent over half the year with lung congestion. The first one went away with all my home remedies and inhalers. The second one I treated like allergies and tried to beat it for four months. After all, we did experience a high pollen count that spring. When I finally went in I was diagnosed with acute bronchitis. I had no other symptoms of being sick: no fever, malaise, loss of appetite. Further tests show I have stage one COPD, but my symptoms more closely resemble stage two. The final exam is coming.

It's almost better, for me, to be dealing with a chronic lung condition. It gives me a sense of purpose. It's imminent, like cramming for a test the day before. Without my medical diagnosis I would be born into a caste of privilege where everyone assumes general health. It gives me impetus for research, where the knowledge gained can be strewn together to form new theories and ideas to slow progression, exercise...buy more time. It creates a fervor of recognizing each day as a gift and taking steps to prolong life. Prior to that, life was a mystery and no one really has any idea when their day will come. We all hope to make it to 100, but like learning new material in the classroom, a pop quiz can appear at any time. What steps did you take to get ready? I've always been a procrastinator even when I knew there was a test coming at the end of the term. I just wasted time by going out to play, watching television and riding my bike. I had nothing to lose in earlier life because I had nothing to live for. I finally got my act together and bought a house, got married, have pets. Now I'm dying. I typically spend 20% of each year drowning or recovering from it. My lungs fill with congestion and it's too deep to cough out. I just cough because I can't breathe. It gives me practice for my final days when this illness prevails over me.

I've also received another important diagnosis that wouldn't have been possible in a prior century. In 1942 Dr Harry Klinefelter identified a syndrome in which men had small testicles, gynecomastia, were tall, often sterile and lacking in secondary sex characteristics. He named it Klinefelter's Syndrome. I think it's kind of pompous to create eponymous conditions. I resent wearing his name in describing my health. It wasn't until 1956 that it was discovered the guys with KS had an extra X chromosome. I typically like to refer to it as XXY, otherwise I feel the syndrome denotes that I somehow belong to Dr. Klinefelter. It was also during the 1950s that longer esters were added to injectable testosterone, a common prescription for those of us with faulty gonads. The esters are a type of oil that allows an injection to last longer by slowly releasing the medicine into the body. Otherwise testosterone has a very short half-life. So, I'm satisfied people like me occupy this place in history. The knowledge and medicine have potential.

Aside from quality of life concerns, I might have fared better as a serf under Feudalism. I tend to live more for the moment under institutionalized circumstances. I thrive in external locus control situations, which means people who attribute their success or failure on outside influences. I've been shown two sides of life: there was me unable to control my antics, always disrupting the class or society and procrastination. Then there was me who was punished and it was through various means of punishment that I learned what works best for me. In-school suspension, prison and being dominated in a relationship are external forms of control in which I become a good person. Feudalism was considered a dominant social system in Medieval Europe, which makes me think I'd do well. There would have been less pollen and fewer people on the planet in the period which spanned from the Early Middle Ages to the mid 19th century. The Industrial Revolution didn't officially begin until 1789 in France, so the act of removing carbon from the earth in order to burn in the atmosphere hadn't made that much of an impact by the 1850s, when Feudalism officially ended. Breathing would have been better and life would have been spent thinking about the here and now, mostly out of poverty and hunger concerns. That sort of control would have made me a better person. On the contrary, in our current free society, my idle mind worries against me. I obsess too much (as if there were a way to obsess in moderation). I'm too free to think about the many health conditions people with XXY face. I'm at risk of developing breast cancer; the same risk as a woman. I get screened for lumps each year by my endocrinologist. My chest development is more similar to that of a female than a male, so I don't go shirtless in public. I worry about fitting in with men and what it means to be masculine.

When I was in my mid-teens, I would masturbate while looking at my breasts in the mirror. I fantasized about being a girl and it turned me on. As I got older I fantasized about being with a man until I finally made the plunge to see what it was about. It was traumatic to experience something that went against how I was raised and the identity I had established. I guess it would be comparable to getting away with having committed a violent crime because you could never talk about it without fear of being in trouble. I just had to live with thinking something was wrong with me and what I needed sexually was considered wrong by all the people I'd ever known.

I've been haunted by a ghost of masculinity. It was a living idea once, but it has been gone longer than I ever thought it pertained to me. Aside from sucking a dick at age 18, knowing I was behaving the way straight women do, what little understanding I had of masculinity was removed from me abruptly at a doctor's appointment. There was no counseling or ways of healing. The news was handed down like a summary execution and I interpreted it as *you are not a man.* Again, I had no one to talk with about it. I would have risked dismantling my character in the eyes of others; their judgment. That doctor told me my testicles were 1/8 the size of normal. As a boy in school, everything was exaggerated as big as everyone joked and bragged. I buried this newfound shame with alcohol and between not feeling masculine and being bisexual, my innermost fears were projected outward. I developed a fascination with men's balls. When a man sits a certain way, I'll sometimes sneak looks at their crotches. I'm so curious how they look naked and what kind of bulge their pants show. I worry that my pants don't show a bulge. I'm perpetually envious of males who've developed normally.

I will sneak looks and glances long after I've been caught and I can't get the urge out of my head. It becomes a compulsion. I become hyper-aware of their tone and body language. I see how their attitude toward me changes. They get visibly upset as if I've violated them and there's nothing I can do to fix it. I'm sure it gives them a sense of homophobia. No one has gone so far as to want to fight or yell at me. Usually it happens while talking with friends. It happened to me in prison and it's happened at work. They typically start making comments and saying things to each other, like inside jokes where I'm to be shamed. I've heard gay and fag references or people just outright avoiding me. I don't blame them. It has cost me friendships.

I've had to lie to all the women I've ever been with about my attraction to men. Many were bisexual themselves. I would float ideas and comments to gauge their response. The women I dated often responded that male on male sex is "nasty" and "unnatural." I've only dated women. I think I would fear being judged in public for being with a man. I wouldn't be able to show affection to him in front of others without fear of disdain by anyone around. I know about the privileged beliefs in the outside world because I am trapped by them. I feel I live as an actor for the benefit everyone else around; complete strangers guide my life.

I've never had a safe environment to be honest about who I was. I kept a part of me in the closet and pretended to be straight for others, to be safe, but also to protect myself from their shitty perspectives. I'm not nasty or unnatural, nor do I deserve abuse for being who I am. I can't change it. I know because I've tried. I didn't choose what I like and I can't answer whether a life of lying was better than coming out. But I do know there's a strange caveat in all this: The women who are most vocal in being anti-gay have undoubtedly slept with people like me.

From the childhood game of fearing those with "cooties" to the awareness of our own bodies, gender expression and later sexuality, new fears emerged. Having all the privilege equates your lifestyle as normal and right. A person whose birth certificate says male and identifies as a male and who is attracted to females has privilege. It's only when you have none are you able to analyze the entire system and realize how primitive it is. The shunning of gays is merely an adaptation of a childish game, but it involves so much shame because of genitalia and sexuality. The degradation mainly affects those whose job it was to uphold the idea of masculinity. If you fell outside the definitions of that box you weren't respected. Words like "fag" and "sissy" were thrown about. Girls who were boyish were dotted as "tomboys" and yet, it wasn't the same sort of scorn boys endured. She got to wear boyish clothes and play games with the boys. Similar to the Nazis whose function was to procure the finest human specimens worthy of life, the patriarchy seeks to groom those who can withstand insults and temptations. They become tough and hardened, which are viewed as qualities. Boys did what they could not to be labeled anything less than masculine and girls avoided those who did. It was a game of hot potato with real consequences. You could be called it whether it was true or not. I grew up to live those roles and secretly share those imaginary gay cooties with women who had that exaggerated fear. It was important for me to blend into straight society and when I had sex with women who had strong anti gay views this reaffirmed my dissociation. I hid in bed with venomous serpents who inevitably had sex with others who shared their beliefs and before you know it, the most hardcore redneck has been connected in the chain of all your sexual partners' partners; he's more or less had sex with a homosexual. When an ex-girlfriend and her new boyfriend are heard being disrespectful toward me, I can just smile.

Men are like a medicine for me. I use them for sex. The urges and cravings build until I need to go out and relieve the pressure. It quenches a craving and goes away for a while. I don't know where it goes, perhaps it haunts someone else. Sometimes it's enough to fix me from staring at crotches, but not always. My staring episodes are one of the barometers I use to indicate that it's time to seek out a homosexual experience. Without it, I could resist my urges and live in disguise longer. I try to manage my neuroticisms by acting out, sexually. I need fresh experiences with large testicles. I get to a point where I miss the beauty. It's like walking away from a mirror. At some point I will need to revisit one for a variety of reasons, even though underneath it all, I still know what I look like.

My shame and homosexual desires are inversely related: when one is high, the other is low. It *is* the relationship between prolactin and testosterone. Before orgasm, testosterone is high and many things sound hot and sexy. After climax, testosterone dips and prolactin spikes. Many of those same dirty ideas no longer seem appealing. Prolactin is my shame hormone. Post-orgasm with a man is when my will to be heterosexual is at its peak. I tell myself: *I'll be better this time.*

I'm still attracted to those feminine features on my body that I discovered as a teenager and I love seeing myself as a woman. I'm an avid crossdresser in private. I've grown to foster her identity when I can. My XXY condition fits under the umbrella term of intersex, which means a person who doesn't fit typical definitions of male or female. I don't know that it makes me a cross dresser or trans because first we'd have to identify which I am to begin with. I'm really both and I enjoy identifying as each, depending on my surroundings. I'm not passable as a female, but then again I worry all the time about trying to pass as a man. Life is all about pretending one way or the other for me. I may never know who I truly am.

I'm married too. She goes out of town once in a while and it is something I look forward to. She's mentioned that she doesn't feel missed while she's away. It's difficult for her. I use the time she's away to remove my mask of Carhartt pants and sweatshirts. I live my life as two genders and two sexualities. It's very difficult to wade through life in a shell to outside eyes, knowing it's not what makes me happy. Our discomfort trades places when she leaves town. I become hyper-relaxed and she worries about whether I love her. I typically wear feminine clothes around the house while she's away, then I change back Sunday afternoon and I always feel depressed and anxious afterward. Mine isn't a question of if she loves me, but why?

I've always been drowning. My identity has been defined by the banks of this stream I sail, while my diagnoses have submerged me in medical literature. It's almost a prophecy to die in such a way (drowning in my lungs). The consumer becomes consumed.

News

We like negative gossip as a society. Me, you, everyone we've ever met has found belonging in sharing personal details about others. Our nightly news programs act similarly as they feed us stories of crime, anger and protest. We absorb the briefings while mirroring the lessons. Humans inherently possess characteristics that will never cease. It's the reason we continue finding similarities between current day and the events of the past. Yet ironically, we try to discourage bullying which is regularly reported on in our nightly segments. These two subjects seem very similar to me. On one hand, a company whose medium reaches households across a region exposes people and ideas who've inflamed others. On the other hand, individuals use information against other individuals to expose and inflame.

A person could be gay, have a particular hairstyle, infrequent bathing habits, bite their fingernails, identify as a gender other than the one assigned them, the list goes on. Every case of bullying represents a microcosm of reported media to a group of people who sometimes don't even know the victim. It's not just reported, but it's repeated in ever creative ways to bring shame upon the recipient, sometimes daily. Meanwhile families watch the news together in their living rooms before fading into their individual lives looking for newsworthy gossip to expose others much the same way.

Much like how a class clown maybe doesn't realize he's crossed the line from being laughed *with* vs being laughed *at,* bullying also crosses a line from being passive gossip to becoming an aggressive weapon. Everyone along the chain gets something out of it. It perversely satisfies our sadistic impulses to unmask the secrets of others. After all, it's news, right? People grow up learning these conflicting values from the culture we are indoctrinated into. There's national news as well as a local version. There are well respected programs that delve deeper into stories, sometimes cornering people to ask pointed questions. It's seen as a service to inform the public. There are awards given in an array of categories for investigative journalism. As a viewer I'm hungry for the next scandal.

The narrative always begins the same. First is a story of wrongdoing. The higher the status of an individual, the more sensational it becomes. When it's not an important person the story can still be appealing because of the position the person is in. Every new detail reveals a potentially more embarrassing, shameful act. *We the people* want more. The courts establish depositions, witness accounts, eventually a trial for the perpetrator. As new details emerge we learn them to converse with those we are close with. It brings sustenance to our lives. We bond vicariously as the story unfolds and we demand justice.

Yet, on a more minuscule scale this same behavior takes place in schools, workplaces, housing communities, recreation facilities etc. People are passing information about others, some real, some fabricated. Others in the line of communication aren't always pleasant. They may feel the need to investigate for further minutiae. Daily, the recipient, in this case the victim, is peppered with scorn. Everything is reported from the words they use to defend themselves to their innocent reactions in trying to downplay or deny the accusations. All of it is dissected in group settings for another day's interactions. A person passing gossip should be held accountable for how everyone down the line acts with the information. If I sold drugs to someone who died of an overdose, I would be liable. Same for bartenders who serve someone until they're drunk and cause injury. In some states two people could rob a store and if a clerk kills one of the robbers, the other robber gets charged with that murder because they were liable for each others' wellbeing during the commission of a crime. It's no different if you expose someone to what might bring them hostility and aggression. You are responsible for the wellbeing of the person you humiliate. I don't fault you for how you've grown up, but I find fault in the system that raised us.

Mass shootings plague our nightly news feeds. Not so surprisingly, it's often perpetrated by the victim of bullying; someone who didn't quite fit in. It's kind of ironic to have these two structures so similar and a person ends their misery from one system while being broadcast on the other. It brings new meaning to *live by the sword, die by the sword.* He sought justice for his outcasting and now leaves survivors to bond in the wake of his own pain. By proxy he teaches them a new way to connect. As an onlooker, I knew nothing of a person's pain until their death was thoroughly investigated by the news. Myself and millions of others absorb his story and disseminate it. I understand and hunger for the next tragedy.

Introspection 3

I've always been in a state of stress. Each X chromosome has 1,100 genes while a Y has 200. An XX woman has about 800 more genes than an XY male, which means I have 1,100 more genes than most males and yet, I was identified as one also. I cannot imagine what it must have been like for my body to try and merge 1,100 extra genes into a body while still trying to support life and health. My stressor was internal.

A National Institutes of Health article published May 21, 2019 titled Cellular Stress Associated with Aneuploidy states: "For organisms whose genomes are carried on multiple chromosomes, aneuploidy encompasses thousands to billions of possible numerical combinations of chromosome numbers. As such, aneuploidy, is not a single genetic state but rather a large repertoire of diverse states." The body does try to regulate itself when there's more than one X by silencing approximately 75% the supernumerary X. That's how nature does it in women, but I don't know if having a Y contradicts the process in any way. It's possible I didn't get a complete inactivation. By having 47 chromosomes while 98% of the population has 46 I cannot rule out anything from being possible. Either way, at least 25% of both my X chromosomes are double dosed and I have a Y crowding in there too. I've talked in my other writings about there being genes on the X chromosome having to do with the immune system. Having a funky dosage of those genes opens up the possibility of autoimmune disorders for those of us with more than one X chromosome. The article I cited above goes on to discuss how cells carrying extra copies of chromosomes would overproduce proteins causing them to misfold. (Think of a chromosome as a shelf with genes on it. Those genes often produce proteins. If there were three sets of a gene on a shelf that typically holds two, there might be over production of certain proteins.) I've found genes in PAR1 and PAR2 groupings that are found in both the X and Y chromosomes - about 29 different genes (so far) have been identified in these groups. In closing, "Several cellular stress states have been observed to be associated with aneuploidy: proteotoxic, metabolic, replication and mitotic." In *Introspection 1* I mentioned how XX individuals may have been predisposed to nurture. The priming I received was in coping. I would have loved to know all this when I was being sent to the principal's office. I would have used it as a get out of jail card: *My proteins are misfolding again. I need to lie down!*

I grew up hypersexual, which was counterintuitive because I didn't get a full puberty and was later diagnosed with a condition where my testosterone is low. I read a study from Sweden's *Karolinska Institutet* published by Science Daily November 2, 2015 that found hypersexual disorder is linked to hyperactive stress systems. I have lots of evidence of stress while growing up: in grade school I chewed my fingernails, disrupted the class, paranoia plagued me for many years, I withdrew from the world into daydreaming and later sexual role play. I think acting out sexually might have just been an adaptation of daydreaming, except it was interactive - I could actually take part in the fantasy, like virtual reality. More parts of it could come true vs thinking about winning the lottery.

The stress hormone cortisol is anti-inflammatory, so if a body had high stress it would also pump out cortisol, which can inhibit both oxytocin (the love hormone) and testosterone. I wouldn't produce much testosterone anyway because of the hypogonadism, but a lack of oxytocin contributes to me not feeling close with others. Not only do my lack of social skills prevent me feeling cohesion with the group, but chemically the barrier exists. I seem to be over-primed for a stress response and under for pro-social interactions. My body and personality were meant to suffer alone and in silence.

Identity

Hypochondriac, boy, girl, intersex, inmate, recovery...Identity is defined as who you are, the way you think about yourself, the way you are viewed by the world and the characteristics that define you. At one point in time I was by definition a man at age 18. By age 19 it was stolen from me. Who would you be if parts of your identity were stripped from you? Could you continue living in the image you had created even though you believed deep down it was a lie?

My journey has revealed many facets of life. I have played the sometimes opposing elements as if I were on a stage, performing for a crowd's approval. My act, however, was not a lead role. I didn't proclaim any character and move forward in its expression to grow *with* the audience. My role was reactionary, in that I played cards that were already dealt. The world stage is full of privilege and I follow behind trying to blend in. If men dress a certain way, I dress that way. I'm an actor taking cues from the audience about my role. It's improv for me.

Several times I've lost the piece of who I thought I was. When all your surroundings disappear, who does it make you? I've had to do it in prison: moving to new units, getting out, going to college and new jobs. I have begun anew at least a dozen times and throughout each of them I used my chameleon-like skills to blend in with the people there, even though they didn't represent who I was. Each new attempt at a different life starts with the same basic premise: that I am a straight man. Yet neither of those components are true.

I've always lived closeted. From toys to clothes, I've had desires to do things typically associated to women since grade school. I had a high pitched voice that I was embarrassed of until the 8th grade. By the 9th grade I had boobs that turned me on enough that I would push them together and masturbate to them in front of a mirror. I experimented with cross dressing and I started having fantasies of being with men. I had feelings of being dumb and sexually inadequate throughout high school. There was always an underlying dysmorphia not far away that was buried in shame. Shortly into adulthood I found out from a doctor that my testicles never matured, which I've always resented. I've resented not being normal and every sexual partner who failed to point it out prior to that visit. What could they have been thinking when things didn't look right? I was later diagnosed with an intersex condition called Klinefelter's Syndrome. Life continued humming at a low monotone and by all appearances I was continuing the charade of being a straight man to all eyes. The older I got the more effort I felt to portray the idea of a man.

The function of testicles is to procreate life: the privilege that humans are capable of reproducing in adulthood. What I carry was sentenced to die before I attained its innate ability. My vessels of creation needed a lifejacket, essentially becoming vessels of deception. Why must I carry them with me? I empty my groceries and don't continue carrying the bag around. The bag is then refuse, or used for such and discarded. I'm no different than a broken machine. Why would you keep it? I've failed to grow into any of the males I looked up to as a child and neither do I resemble the females. I am an outsider.

The word genitalia brings to my mind the word tail. Penis is actually derived from a Latin word for tail. It reduces me to the animal kingdom where I have a tail in the front. Mates in other species are attracted to markings, wings, dominance, scent, with an emphasis in human culture on front tails. The etymology of genitalia, however, means reproductive organs. I'm sterile, so what do I have? If I showed it in public it would be described in police reports as genitalia - to box me in with others who have similar parts, but technically there's no ability to use it for reproduction. It excretes liquid waste. It's a tool, an apparatus, a medical device and most of all it's an "it," unworthy of being grouped with functional reproductive organs.

I've lived in denial about the things I liked as if they were manageable or could be bargained away. I've feared being labeled a sexual deviant, so I got my needs met in private or through masturbation. It took me years of doing the same things over and over and getting the same results before I realized it was a part of my identity, albeit a secret one. I felt shame over my desires and the stigma of who it made me. I lived in contempt; life was one way, yet my actions were another. Who was I? I was a male who enjoyed being with other males on occasion. But I was closeted about it and lived dissociated between my public self vs my private self.

Ego is defined as a person's self-esteem, self-importance or self-worth. I had none of those things after learning about my empty, infantile testicles. It challenged my ability to engage with others and I never quite fit in with the normal crowds. There's too much faking that goes into passing as just a regular guy and I'm not that good. I try my best to portray myself as straight + man and I always wonder if either of those are believed. The things that catch me up the most in trying to come off as normal are: eye contact, reacting appropriately to what was said and feeding a conversation. I have a lot on my mind during conversations with men and women, especially those who intimidate me. I desperately try not to get caught being anything other than the man they think they're talking to. But shame has made me timid, fearful, sad and full of guilt. I am a ball of negative emotions that drive inward. I'm afraid of being caught and exposed as a fraud. Feminist author and professor, bell hooks (she does not capitalize her name), writes: "*The first act of violence that patriarchy demands of males is not violence toward women. Instead patriarchy demands of all males that they engage in acts of psychic self-mutilation, that they kill off the emotional parts of themselves. If an individual is not successful in emotionally crippling himself, he can count on patriarchal men to enact rituals of power that will assault his self-esteem.*" Men are supposed to be rough, emotionless, strong etc. I'm none of those things. I worry about upsetting people or them being upset with me. I'm always looking for clues of people's intent and it has caused difficulties in social settings.

I can't really talk to men and I've had a lifelong fear of judgment from women, yet most frequently, it's a certain type of woman I seem to find that I can open up to. I don't know if they're the women I wish I was or if they sense I'm feminine. I'm almost predatory in my pursuits to find them. I look for softness and understanding. I value safety and it is only in the presence of these angels that I feel secure in my being. I've been able to work through trauma by trusting and though it doesn't always resolve my conflict, I'm able to at least disclose personal information and fears. I find people who I can come out to and it frees me from having to wear a burdensome shield. I despise having to live up to hyper-inflated masculine expectations. I don't want to fill a masculine role because I will fail. My trust in disclosure is a way of managing the part of my identity in how others perceive me. I feel they need to know I'm not "him," whoever it is they see across from them. I'm tall and muscular. But I am not him. He died at a doctor's appointment during the mid-nineties. It's strange to go from feeling the thorns of humanity to finding roses among them. I'm relieved to find these islands of safety on the rocky rapids I travel. Without them I wouldn't be able to face a life that's constantly throwing people at me who have ideas on who a man is and how he's supposed to act.

I had always met people and became friends with those I liked. When I started dating my wife I got along great with her adult children but it didn't quite feel the same as the friends I'd always acquired in life. To them, at least one, I was filling a role. I felt the friendship was somewhat standoffish. I was dating a parent and to some degree I was seen as something other than a friend. I couldn't just be a human who liked another human. There were strings attached to these new associates. It was a foreign feeling for me to have this friend who didn't behave the way my friends always had. Dating someone was enough to alter people's perceptions of me even though I was the same person I had always been.

A game I like to play in certain company is similar to a ping that a computer sends to a server. When the ping is sent back, it's an indication that the network is connected. What I do is send out an undercover ping: I will send out toxic comments to see what kind of toxins I receive back. It lets me test what kind of people I'm around and whether I can relax or remain guarded. In my younger years I projected a dislike of gays to see if people would agree with me. But as I've gotten older I just bring up the topic of homosexuality or transgender. Perhaps an artist or musician, something in the recent news. If people are going to be shitty I let them initiate the mood. It brings suspicion on me to have irrational fears and anger about homosexuality and I've learned to blend in better than that. I became better at hiding; a change from the mask of heterosexuality to a more covert display. Even my false identities undergo change from time to time. Who am I?

I've never realized my full potential. I only find belonging in writing about the pain in my life. You as the reader consume it and somehow I fit in, but because of the foundation, I have to go out and hurt more so I can continue writing this thing we share.

Tides

I noticed her name tag, Cara, as I was daydreaming through the formalities. She measured my blood pressure, oximeter on my finger and thermometer in my mouth. I was thinking I could write and publish letters to each of them or set up a fund that bought something nice each year for their offices. I make visits to healthcare clinics so frequently that it is my comfort zone. I'm no longer nervous about whatever news awaits me. I'm so at ease that I take time to read their name tags and appreciate their kindness.

Cara had me perform a lung function test. There was a tube that led into a mouthpiece. It was wired to a laptop, which displayed a simulation of candles on a birthday cake. She instructed me to exhale and point the mouthpiece in the direction of all the candles to blow them out. I've been congested over half the year and I'm used to breathing with only the top half of my lungs. Blowing through the tube caused me to lose the bulk of my air within 1-2 seconds. I timed myself, finding it took an additional 14 seconds to exhale the bottom half, so to speak, of the air trapped inside me. I was pushing a steady stream of air out as I was in need of more coming in. I continued pushing as the last pockets of air bubbled through my congestion. I completed the simulation three times and I never got all the candles out.

My situation is spelled out to me clear as day. Every few years I gain a new medication or inhaler. This year I had bronchitis in the summer and it took two rounds of different antibiotics. In addition, I was on prednisone for 10 days. Today at my appointment inCara's office I was prescribed Symbicort. The doctor wants me to use it in place of Qvar, which I am to use when my lungs are acting up. Except he told me to use Symbicort twice per day whether I felt I needed it or not. A person could read this a couple different ways. It is a different drug, perhaps it works best to build up in the system; it requires daily use. Or, perhaps my condition is worsening and I require not only a stronger medication, but one all the time.

I'm essentially on life support, only it's under very favorable terms. It fits in my pocket and no one even has a suspicion. I'm not weighed down with an oxygen tank or connected to an IV. I was given a prescription for a nebulizer for use during illness. When I called the company that supplies such equipment, their automated phone system asked me to press digits to speak with certain departments. One of the divisions dealt with hospice care. These subtle hints help normalize my advancing demise. By the time I need hospice equipment I will already have an account with a company that deals in death. I also use a CPAP which adds an interesting dynamic - I'm connected to a breathing apparatus for 8 hours per night. I have portable inhalers throughout the day and a nebulizer for times of illness. Do the machines represent life or death, as I slowly require more time with them? I accept new prescriptions in ever increasing strength to ease my suffering. Each new medication plays the dual role escorting death inside me while chaperoning my body to allow the transition.

Trained medical personnel observing my vital signs have assigned me as alive. Numerous dictionaries define alive as meaning *not dead.* I could argue against what they've told me. During an active flare up when I awaken unable to breathe and my coughing is uncontrollable, I wonder about my own designation: *life.* I'm neither alive nor dead. In those moments of grasping for life, I am the quintessential Shrodinger's cat. *Trans* meaning across, I'm mixed between the two and it is only through medical intervention that I'm propped up as a puppet to fit their definition of life. I'm transdeath and it's a scam to sell equipment so I can jump through the hoops that certify me a certain way. Each time I reach a new pinnacle for care, the cost goes up. My Symbicort inhaler, that they want me to use daily, costs $70. Without insurance, it's $393. They get their exorbitant fees because they're selling hope.

When I went on road trips as a child I remember all the splattered bugs on the windshield. We'd have to ask the gas station attendant to clean it. As an adult the bug populations have been in a steady decline. Rarely is it an issue to need dead bugs cleaned from the glass. My issue now is more complex as it requires cleaning the inside of my windshield from all the splotches left from a season's worth of coughing. In a twist of irony my lungs are cleaning themselves as my windshield becomes dirtier and it's exponentially more difficult to clean the inside than the out.

Link

I've been reading that scientists are finding a link between gut bacteria and autism in their hunt to understand it. Diagnosed cases have gone up in recent years, though it is not a new condition. Asperger's is actually named after an Austrian pediatrician. During WWII this sick fuck noticed a group of kids who had an extraordinary ability to learn and recall information. They were spared while the others who didn't possess such abilities were sent off to be murdered. He didn't actually name it after himself. It wasn't until 1981 that someone wrote a paper and referenced his name.

In the 1960s and 70s, autism was reported in the US and Europe at a rate of about 2-4 per ten thousand. It was during the cold war, so it's likely that some of our official data was skewed to try and reflect a "healthy" population. I use that in quotes because it doesn't reflect my language. I'm only putting myself in the perspective of Cold War censors who were fighting an informational war with the Soviet Union. They might have wanted to show we were more perfect than other nations. Today diagnoses for autism are at an astounding 1 in 59 or 169 in ten thousand. Reasons could be our doctors are trained better. Our population has grown by 50% since 1970 so there are more of us and more doctors. There's a night and day difference in medical textbooks from the aforementioned era compared to the ones of today. Or maybe there's something from our lifestyles contributing to it.

The top 5 countries for autism are US, Japan, Canada, UK, Ireland. Those are all industrialized economies. The next 5 include Brazil and Portugal as nine and ten respectively. This leads me to believe it's something environmental, but what could affect our gut bacteria? The obvious answer is food, either something in it or how it was raised/grown.

People often blame vaccines and I'm totally against that idea. I even get a flu shot every year. I want more vaccines, like 3 strains of flu every month. When a coronavirus vaccine comes out, I'm getting it as well. I think what people are looking for is something that affects all of us. If we find it, that's our link. For them, it's vaccinations. I've read where some people theorize the sound from a sonogram might be as loud as a train to a baby and they think that could be it. It could also be a byproduct of the Industrial Revolution in the air we breathe or the water we drink.

Do we look for the reason why it has ever existed or do we just look for why the numbers seem to have increased? My theory is centered around antibiotic use. Penicillin was first discovered in 1928. It wasn't until the mid-late 1940s that antibiotics were prescribed to the general population. In 1950 it was discovered that adding them to the feed of livestock accelerated growth and profit. The reason, at least in cows, was they naturally eat grass, which has bacteria on it. This helps to ferment their meal to unlock all its nutrients and the process can take several days. Farmers found that feeding their cattle grains can speed up the process, but the lack of digestive enzymes and fiber caused ulcers and buildup of harmful bacteria like Clostridium perfringens or E. coli. These can create obsesses and leak into other organs, even causing sudden death of the cow. The trick should have been to keep them healthy until it made it to your dinner plate, instead it was merely to keep them alive and gaining weight. It came down to the bottom dollar, greed and artificially speeding up a natural process. Whether your family ate healthy beef or not was not the top concern. I found an article on CNN while researching this that said farmers were feeding candy to cows in 2012 because the price of corn was so high.

Antibiotics wipe out your gut bacteria - the good and the bad. Think about the fact that we've essentially been eating sick animals for 70 years. At the very least they were sick because they didn't have adequate levels of gut bacteria. Many including penicillin, work by attacking the wall of a bacteria's cell. Others inhibit cell walls from being made (vancomycin). Still, others shut down vital parts of microbial reproduction, protein synthesis or development of RNA. We assume everything grows back in time, but do we really know if it all comes back or in the ratios as was natural? The original antibiotic was grown from mold. If your body senses that you have eaten mold, it's going to try and defend against it. Even though what we make now is manufactured in a lab, it still behaves the same way. Biologically, our bodies have evolved to recognize molecular effects. Examples of this idea are the myriad of carbs and sugars now on store shelves that didn't exist 100 years ago. When we eat them, our bodies still recognize them as sugars and carbs even though they were created in a lab. What's also interesting is that vaccines contain small amounts of antibiotics. It's in there to keep the serum from molding and spoiling. There's also a trace amount of mercury, called thiomersal. It's in there to act as an antifungal. Like I've said, I'm not an "anti-vaxxer." I'm just looking for a link.

Camps

If the Holocaust were happening today many of you would be working in camps. Not forced, you would actually leap for the opportunity to blindly serve your country. At that time all world economies were in a depression and Germany was working toward prosperity. You think you'd rather sit and starve? Easy to say in hindsight. Even the slave laborers fed their own family and friends into the furnaces in order to prolong their lives another day. Everyone took part in the annihilation of "undesirables," erasing those who'd been hated for hundreds of years.

Jewish chemist and Holocaust survivor Primo Levi said "It happened, therefore it could happen again." The fact that humans worked in the camps means that you, as a human, have as much integrity to rationalize whatever job you would be assigned: "I was only guarding, I was only doing roll call, I was only escorting the sick and weak to the showers. I was only following orders."

I say everyone because even those who passively ignored the machine working around them were guilty. I'm no different. In prison there were groups of people we all had to hate regardless of their personalities. It wasn't in my best interest to buck the system and befriend an "undesirable." All it would do is make me also an undesirable. I know enough about history, human nature and myself to admit that I, too, have the potential to go along with the masses.

With our current political situation, there's more transparency than there was during the Holocaust. I can disagree without fear of bucking the system. I can band with others and create an opposition that's strong enough that others can find us and feel safe. I choose not to hate, we choose not to hate.

I want a professional in my next president who can be quiet on occasion. I want a person with their own ideas and who doesn't mock their enemies. Remember when John McCain stuck up for his opponent rather than ride a wave of hatred? That's what I want. I don't want someone who speaks with chants of hatred from his audience. I've seen enough black and white clips on YouTube from an earlier time when people chanted. The bonding that comes with hatred is a strong force. In my opinion, it is more powerful than bonding via greatness. I'd rather feel prideful in lifting up those around me than in boosting my sense of self by stepping on those deemed undesirable. I need someone who can be accountable and not place blame.

We've had no shortage of enemies these last few years. I've seen friends in Kansas who hate a congresswoman in New York. Yet I doubt they can name any previous NY Congress members; they only know the names of those who've opposed our projector in chief. The person in the pulpit is a laser. When dissent is raised, the subsequent wrath is a concentrated beam of attack, a blitzkrieg if you will. A name not widely known today: Herschel Feibel Grynszpan. He was used as a catalyst to advance an agenda in a bygone era. He was Polish born Jew living in France who watched his rights as an immigrant erode and his family rounded up and deported. He lashed out and assassinated a German diplomat in Paris. After a couple days the young junior diplomat succumbed to his injuries on November 9. Having met with the German leader, Goebbels wrote in his diary: "The Jews should feel the people's fury." That night is now known as Kristallnacht.

November 9th, 2016, marked our own descent into chaos. I can't even name the top 3, 5 or 10 most bat shit crazy things spoken by our President since then. He seems to bend reality when he speaks as well as assail the English language. We have lists of states, countries and nationalities who've suffered. I don't share any of the fury against these groups he's labeled "enemies." I read a meme that said: If illegals are freeloaders, why does ICE always raid workplaces? Another said: If you think that Mexico is only sending drug dealers and rapists, but also worry they're going to take your job, what the fuck do you do for a living? I seek logic from a leader.

I want a person who doesn't have an 80+% turnover rate for their cabinet positions and I want the workers in those posts to feel safe, to feel validated by their ideas and objections, to not only do what's legal, but to also do what's moral and in the interest of all Americans. I want policies that serve the nation and its allies. I want the opposite of what I have now. I'm looking for an element that used to live here, named truth.

Take a look around and note who the Trump supporters are. He appeals largely to people from dysfunctional backgrounds. Some day they'll be released from his spell, his constant interruptions to our lives. Each and every one of his misstatements serves a polarizing purpose. It agitates his enemies and doses his proponents like medicine. It doesn't matter how flamboyant are his lies. It's his purpose to stay relevant; to keep them drunk and under his influence. I dated a girl who did this very thing to me. Once I was able to separate from the madness, pieces of reality set in. The more we stayed a part the more it all made sense and I vowed to recognize the red flags that showed again in someone else. Pay attention to who you see in your life that endorses Trump. They are similarly sick. I don't know if they'll ever see the light and recognize it for what it is. I do know they don't share our humanity toward one another and I don't care what their point of support is. Even those who wanted a better tax system are excusing and pardoning cruelty. These friends of ours are not allies of compassion.

I want my next President to restore employment and reputation to those who've lost on America's latest domestic battlefield: James Comey, Richard Spencer, James Mattis, Col Vindman, captain Khan, John McCain, Robert Mueller... (That list is quite long) But I also want Andrew McCabe to receive his full retirement.

I need a President who'll do what's right. As leader of the free world I'm looking for someone who doesn't take a vacation every weekend and doesn't fight to the Supreme Court to hide his taxes after telling us he'd release them. I'm conducting interviews up until November 2020.

3 Minutes of Courage

It's routine for me to collect supplies as I need them. I order and stockpile until the day it's needed. It's kept in a drawer in a spare bedroom. I gather them together once in a blue moon and contemplate something seemingly inescapable. I can't help but question my being. I'm always in a dark and heavy depression by the time I unite the items from my hidden cache.

That's how it's been over the last few years. I've started questioning many things in life. I consume medical literature to try and understand this or that. Each piece of knowledge that I gain subtracts from my identity. Intellectually, I'm sinking in quicksand. I've become hyper-aware of people like me, yet nescient of who I am. I live in a prison, slave to a synthetic self.

I use testosterone. My body doesn't really make it and because I have a penis it was prescribed to help to assist my body in being healthy like men are supposed to be. For those same reasons, estrogen wasn't a talk worth having. I've never even had my estrogen levels tested because my endocrinologist sees "no reason." Forget that there are other symptoms like breasts or that I have the genetic makeup of both a man and a woman. My own body was so confused by the conflicting data that it failed to mature my testicles beyond the size of childhood. A penis seems to outweigh any other evidence for a counter argument, so a doctor gets to decide it's an easier fit for me to be male. Testosterone modified my body into what cisgendered men probably strive for in outwardly appearance. Modify is defined as - make partial or minor changes to (something), typically so as to improve it or to make it less extreme. My body has been modified with the help of science. Synthetic hormones are the crutch I use to stagger a simulated man through life.

I don't know if I'm trans because I don't know what I am. Am I a woman who has a penis or am I a male with female features? If my skeleton were found by anthropologists, I would most definitely be identified as a female because of my hips. It doesn't seem like they can do chromosome tests on skeletons, but even then, could they reach a conclusion? The Smithsonian channel did a piece recently on a high ranking soldier from the

Revolutionary War, Casimir Pulaski. The thinking is that this person was intersex because their hips were wide and had delicate facial bones. Perhaps I'm trans by default because our binary system only identifies one or the other, so whichever one I am, I'm also the other. Ask Mr. Trump which bathroom I should use.

I doubt I would have taken estrogen at the time of my diagnosis even if it were offered. I was still thinking I could make it as a man way back then. I was in a male prison at the time so I needed steroids to get big. It was my ticket to escape into a new role while my surroundings remained constant. I've always struggled to make negligible decisions, let alone life changing resolutions. I tend to stay in my routine out of familiarity. I had no idea where I'd be today with my identity and still, I may continue where I am rather than risk change. My life is based on being a man. I continue, free in society, but still in a man's prison.

I was wanting to create a word that meant self-prison. That's what my shot has become to me. I was looking at *sui* meaning one's own self, taken from suicide and Medieval Latin *penalis* for penal. But I don't know what rules would apply ie; dropping i to add an e in creating an English word from two Latin words. *Suipenalis* doesn't roll off my tongue easily, but maybe the foreign feel is because it has never existed until now. In my hunt I found *ignosco* which is Latin for pardon, which is equally deep in the sense that my shot is a pardon from a sentence that began from my last shot. My next shot will pardon this current one, but begins a new penance.

I draw up my syringe using a 19 gauge needle because of testosterone's thickness. It is a syrupy liquid like. Once my syringe reaches my prescribed dosage, I remove the needle from the vial and detach it from the syringe. I then place a smaller 23 gauge, 1 ½" needle to inject it into my buttocks. I do this because I don't like to insert a needle into my body which has already penetrated a rubber stopper. I prefer a fresh, smaller needle. Sometimes I'll shoot it into my shoulder out of laziness and ease of use. The courage to poke myself is really short in duration. I'm in my 40s, but I don't need to gather 40+ years of cumulative strength. I just need courage for about a minute or less to drive the steel straw into my body. Within a few hours probably 90% of my depressed feelings are gone. I am a transformer, reshaping from a crumpled sad mess to a masculine being who craves sex. I could keep the depression away more if I used it regularly, but I have reasons for avoiding it. If I dosed myself weekly, I would probably get depressed a little more than the average person, but wouldn't necessarily be as deep. I regularly withdraw and it's almost as if I enjoy my depressive contemplations.

In the beginning I used testosterone almost religiously and coupled it with a weightlifting program. I grew and ate and reveled in the attention I got from my hard work. I would elicit a room's attention as I made my entrance. I became something I had never been before and it showed a different side to life. Eventually my routine died off in sections. The first thing to go was my exercise routine, then my diet and I developed a gut. Work and bills became my primary focus.

I've always had a fascination with researching my condition. In the beginning it was outdated encyclopedias and medical textbooks that all had the same generic information. Our prison library was limited to old, donated books. I think most every book on the subject from 1960-1990 was written from the same general press release. Once free, I advanced to college libraries to read about gender differences in the brain and development. I'd read studies on hormones and the effects of animals receiving opposite sex hormones. One such study looked at male mice that were castrated neonatally, then administered estrogen around puberty. It showed the male mice behaved like females, in lordosis, which is the posture of females being mounted by males.

That's how I identify with my own story. I've never made ideal levels of testosterone. My testicles have never matured. As far as volume is concerned, they are about 3 ml, or the size of a grape. On top of that deficiency, people with my condition have been known to express hyperestrogenism. What that means is having an increase in the activity by which males create estrogen: aromatase. It's my theory that the little bit of testosterone I do make gets converted into estrogen at a higher rate than is typical for males. I am that castrated mouse behaving as a female.

It brings me shame because I was conditioned otherwise while growing up. Most people identify with the gender they were assigned at birth; the one delivery room doctors believe aligns with one's genitalia. I was pronounced a boy and my parents expected me to be one. There were words among my peers that had traversed generations that kept everyone in their respective boxes: fag and sissy were terms no boy sought to be labeled. Yet, I've always had other desires while pretending to be straight and masculine.

We all start as a female embryo until 6-8 weeks. That's when a gene on the Y chromosome signals a change to occur. The gonads begin in the place where ovaries normally are. In males they move down to become testicles and reside in the scrotum, which forms by the labia fusing together. For me, the physical process happened and I was born a healthy boy -by sight.

During the testosterone surge from the newly organized testicles, brain development is taking place. A boy's brain differentiates in ways concerning volume and areas of gray and white matter. Men have been shown to perform differently than women on certain tasks. MRI scans also show differences. People like me show entirely different on tests and scans. Neither as men or women. I'm somewhere in the middle. No one in the delivery room could have seen whether my testicles functioned correctly or not, not with their eyes. It just takes a little blood to do a karyotype to check for normal chromosome arrangement. I'm curious why we strive for technology that we often fail to utilize.

My particular issue didn't become physically symptomatic until puberty, but I wasn't alerted to it until after high school during a physical. It has led to personal discoveries to help me rationalize the way I am.

I get confused trying to learn new tasks, especially things that men traditionally excel in. Because of my appearance as a man I'm assumed to know certain things and when I don't I feel embarrassed. Mechanical aptitude is not natural for me. When a new task requires more than one step or it doesn't make sense to me, I get frustrated easily. I want to quit and hide. Guys with my condition, Klinefelter's Syndrome, often suffer from learning disabilities. I frequently feel clumsy no matter how strong my will to succeed is. My hands tremor as it is, but when I'm trying not to fail it happens more so and inevitably creates failure on some level.

I like men and women sexually. I also fear the judgement of straight men and all women. Women are intimidating to me, yet I prefer their company once I find the ones I can trust. I'm closeted about my sexuality. First I feared acting on my desires, but then I feared being caught or others finding out after the fact. Instead, I choose to pretend to be straight and hide parts of my past. I've dissociated between who I am and what I pretend to be. I've had several bisexual girlfriends who expressed it being gross for two men to get together. There's a double standard in many circles where it is actually encouraged for women, but only if they're both feminine in appearance. It is seen as a performance for the male ego. These egos don't even see the irony in that they are using a version of gay sex to get off. I have fucked up theories on why I've attracted so many women who were partial to other women, basically because maybe I'm not as virilized as males typically are. I'm like the best of both worlds to them: personality of a woman and plumbing of a male. I also am attracted to transgender women who are pre-op down below. To me, it is the best of both worlds: it keeps me on the side of heterosexuality with the addition of a penis to play with. But also I identify most with her because I feel I am her.

Being submissive to women excites me more than trying to be dominant. I didn't pick what I like and I've tried to break from it because the majority of women I've been with have had needs of their own to be submissive. I look the part of domineering and it must be a disappointment for them to learn otherwise. With men, I prefer to be on the receiving end - I want to be the woman. Even when watching heterosexual porn I focus on being the woman. I notice every piece of beauty on a woman either on film or out in public. From her nails to her eyebrows, shoes, stature etc. I often want to be her or have some attribute. I envy women and want to be one in an effort to escape my current role expectations.

I feel the clothes I wear to work that match my assigned gender are a costume. It's like the guy who wears a Scooby-Doo outfit **every** Halloween. His friends know what to expect and it's a gag for him to portray a cartoon dog. I also wear a silly costume and every day it is my Halloween. My costume comes with a strict acting routine where I cannot afford to slip up. It's not always who I want to be though. My costume is a prison. Conversely, a woman can dress feminine or not. Her mannerisms aren't as restricted. The worst outcome she faces is to be labeled a tomboy, but there aren't any friendly, widely accepted terms for males who fall outside of the box of masculinity.

I fight using my testosterone by skipping it for weeks at a time until whatever horny feeling I have wanes. It's not just my sexualized feelings I fight, it's about being the man that chemistry makes me. I resent "him." Each time I withdraw from the science kit prescribed to me the pretend man in me dies. I have a certain amount of dysphoria with my genitals. The root word of *dys* means bad, hard. Added to *pherein* meaning to carry. *Dysphoria* was coined in English in 1842 to mean "impatience under affliction." I have no patience left in waiting for Priapus[2]. As difficult as it is to carry, "it" accompanies me throughout life, always there, always keeping the acrimony secret. My life becomes just going to work and home and back again. I rarely take time to enjoy the company of others. I couldn't even tell you three things I enjoy doing. I've spent my weekends at home not talking to another soul. It makes something as simple as going to the store a weird feeling. I go from complete solitude to surrounded by people, perhaps the clerk talks *to* me and I feel so lost and out of place. At work I could talk *with* people my entire shift, never mind that I don't always like them. Socializing is important and work provides a form of it already baked into my schedule.

Sometimes I read WW II history when I've had my fill of medical information. I get deep into reading actual documents the Nazis kept. One time I wanted to know who made the crematorium ovens and I spent a weekend reading about a company called Topf and Sons (that's the English translation), who were complicit in the genocide. One member of the family applied for a patent for a 3 story self-fueled crematorium because Auschwitz-Birkenau could never keep up with the demand. They killed as many as ten thousand every day and still wanted more capacity. I always have more questions than the generic information in history books; it's my backup subject. Sometimes I can break from medical research for up to 3 weeks. But then I'm right back reading it. It's definitely a neurosis that takes over my every spare moment. I just search and scour the web looking for answers. Another subject I use is psychology to help me process who I am or how to accept what has happened. Theories on cognitive dissonance, ego, development etc. I like reading about Carl Jung, Michel Foucault, Abraham Maslow...the lists of influencers are as long as the questions I always have.

My reading habits would probably induce depression in the happiest of people. Try consuming intense subjects all weekend, then returning to work for casual conversation: *"What did you do this weekend?"* My go-to answer is that I ran errands and relaxed. I'm not about to admit that I just spent the last 72

---

[2] Priapus -rustic god of fertility, protection of livestock, fruit plants, gardens, and male genitalia

hours researching the psychosocial impact of males with small genitals or the health concerns of those with trisomies or even Nazi war atrocities. Working gives me a place to go to get out of my head. Without it, I would feel less complete.

I'm always carrying a burden. I'm defensively guarding secrets from what I do in my spare time to my past. Questions always seem to arise and when I talk: my history doesn't involve taking motors apart, using tools, which sports team I like, when deer season starts. I fear straight men will suspect I'm not one of them and women will sense I'm not who I appear, even in casual conversation. I even fear using urinals because there I am, exposing my darkest burden. Rationally I know no one at a urinal could see my balls, but I'm not rational in keeping my secrets private.

The prefrontal cortex, which handles logical reasoning, doesn't mature in formation until around age 25. Your amygdala processes emotions which trigger fight/flight/freeze. The two areas communicate with each other, but don't function at the same time. In a highly charged situation, you only get emotional or logical responses, not both. It's the reason an angry person punches holes in the wall. A person's neural pathway strengthens no different than any muscle. People who regularly become enraged do so progressively and I've often read of domestic abusers who go from punching walls to people, eventually killing their lovers. I can apply that same knowledge to my own life and realize the fear response in using the bathroom around others is strong. Things have to be set up just right for me to go: not too many people, partitions, evenly spaced, a little noise, no one talking to me. Each time I avoid it out of fear it becomes more difficult the next time. When I reflect back on it, the only logical answer I have is how irrational the expectation is that I bare a part of my anatomy that I've spent my entire life trying to conceal.

Usually around my 5th or 6th week of abstaining from testosterone, I get depressed. I get in a heavy, dark depression. Biologically I'm withdrawing from testosterone, but internally the "man" is dying and my obsessive reading material drives me lower, yet my thirst for information intensifies as if I find joy in feeling so low. I read to feel free, yet I read to stay isolated. The secrets I'm hiding create stress, yet I'm learning about myself, adding more secrets and I begin to think about all the people who've intersected my life. I wonder how each of them would respond to my suicide and would they understand my looking for freedom from my *suipenalis*. I can easily cry at the thoughts of my closer companions having to deal with it. It's mostly a mental list of my closest coworkers and family members. I resist being a man until my depression reaches its full capacity. I can usually go in that state for about a month after the depression hits, sometimes longer. I could end it one of two ways: On the one hand I could continue subscribing to my counterfeit biology, or I could cease all the madness once and for all and it shouldn't compound the courage I'm acquainted to facing. I could easily end all my internal conflict, my failure to relate to both sexes, learning new tasks, secrets of my personality, I could crumble my entire facade and release all my burdens in one fell swoop, if you will.

I could gather supplies while going back and forth to work. Nothing extraordinary has to happen in the background. Currently when I run out of syringes I order more. When my testosterone runs out, the pharmacy contacts the doctor. I just pick up each piece and put it in the drawer. I could just as easily plan to eat spaghetti on Saturday and gather the ingredients as I go about my week. I think I could peripherally gather other supplies no differently. I could acquire the parts for a final *ignosco*; one that would need no other pardon. And I wouldn't need a lifetime of courage to end a lifetime of despair. The parts could be assembled and used in just a few minutes. There is no difference in piercing my body with a piece of steel, whether it be straw-like or solid. The courage that is needed is small in comparison to its impact.